D1037205

SCOPE and STANDARDS
of
Nursing Informatics
Practice

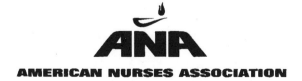
WITHDRAWN FROM
WILLIAM F. MAAG LIBRARY
YOUNGSTOWN STATE UNIVERSITY

ANA

AMERICAN NURSES ASSOCIATION

Washington, D.C.

WILLIAM F. MAAG LIBRARY
YOUNGSTOWN STATE UNIVERSITY

Library of Congress Cataloging-in-Publication Data

Scope and standards of nursing informatics practice.
    p. ; cm.
Includes bibliographical references.
    ISBN 1-55810-166-7
    1. Nursing informatics—Standards.
    [DNLM: 1. Medical Informatics—standards. 2. Nursing—standards. 3.
Medical Records Systems, Computerized. 4. Nursing—organization &
administration. 5. Nursing Records—standards. WY 26.6 S422 2001]
    I. American Nurses Association
    RT50.5 .S36 2001
    610.73′0285—dc21

                                                                    2001045885

Published by
American Nurses Publishing
600 Maryland Avenue, SW
Suite 100 West
Washington, D.C. 20024-2571

©2001 American Nurses Association. All rights reserved.

First printing Oct. 2001. Second printing May 2002.

ISBN 1-55810-166-7

NIP21   2M   03/04R

ACKNOWLEDGMENTS

American Nurses Association Workgroup to Review and Revise the *Scope of Practice for Nursing Informatics and the Standards of Nursing Informatics*

Nancy Staggers, PhD, RN, FAAN, Chairperson

Carole A. Gassert, PhD, RN, FAAN, FACMI

Jan Lee Kwai, MSN, RN,BC, CNOR

D. Kathy Milholland Hunter, PhD, RN

Ramona Nelson, PhD, RN,BC

Joyce Sensmeier, MS, RN,BC

Diane Struck, Lt Col (USAF), MS, RN,BC

John Welton, PhD, RN

ANA Staff

Carol Bickford, PhD, RN,BC

Winifred Carson, JD

Yvonne Humes, BA

The authors are very grateful to Judith Graves, PhD, RN, FAAN, for providing her insights and wisdom that enriched our discussions in the metastructure section of this document.

iii

CONTENTS

INTRODUCTION

Nursing informatics is a specialty that integrates nursing science, computer science, and information science to manage and communicate data, information, and knowledge in nursing practice. Nursing informatics facilitates the integration of data, information, and knowledge to support patients, nurses, and other providers in their decision-making in all roles and settings. This support is accomplished through the use of information structures, information processes, and information technology.

The goal of nursing informatics is to improve the health of populations, communities, families, and individuals by optimizing information management and communication. This includes the use of technology in the direct provision of care, in establishing effective administrative systems, in managing and delivering educational experiences, in supporting life-long learning, and in supporting nursing research.

The purpose of this document is to delineate the scope of nursing informatics practice and the standards for the Informatics Nurse Specialist (INS). However, some sections of this work have application to the informatics needs of all nurses. This document expands on earlier work within nursing informatics (NI), providing historical as well as state-of-the-science material for the specialty (ANA, 1994, 1995). Because of the rapid changes in nursing, computer, and information sciences, NI role specifications, and thinking within informatics, a new document was needed. This revision provides new sections on metastructures and concepts underpinning NI, human–computer interaction, and ergonomics concepts; the evolution of NI definitions; a definition, goal, and role specification for NI; informatics competencies and the roles of the informatics nurse specialist; ethics in nursing informatics; and revised standards of practice.

This revised scope and standards document can be useful in several ways. First, the document outlines the attributes and definition of the specialty, differentiating it from other nursing specialties and validating NI as a distinct specialty within nursing. Second, the document can be useful to informatics educational

vii

programs and NI practitioners as a reference and guide. Third, this work can serve as a reference for employers; for example, to assist with developing of position descriptions. Last, the material can serve as a source document for funding agencies and others seeking to understand NI.

SCOPE OF PRACTICE OF NURSING INFORMATICS

Nursing Informatics

Nursing informatics (NI) is one example of a discipline-specific informatics practice within the broader category of health informatics. NI has become well established within nursing since its recognition as a specialty for registered nurses by the American Nurses Association (ANA) in 1992.

The specialty of NI is important to nursing and health care. It focuses on the representation of nursing data, information, and knowledge (Graves and Corcoran, 1989; Henry, 1995) and the management and communication of nursing information within the broader context of health informatics. Nursing informatics (1) provides a nursing perspective, (2) illuminates nursing values and beliefs, (3) denotes a practice base for nurses in NI, (4) produces unique knowledge, (5) distinguishes groups of practitioners, (6) focuses on the phenomena of interest for nursing, and (7) provides needed nursing language and word context (Brennan, 1994) to health informatics.

Specialty Attributes of Nursing Informatics

Panniers and Gassert (1996), who applied Styles' (1989) earlier work on specialization to informatics, discussed the following five attributes or characteristics that must be present to designate a specialty in nursing:

- A differentiated practice
- A defined research program
- Organizational representation
- Educational programs
- A credentialing mechanism

Differentiated Practice

The focus of nursing informatics (NI) separates or differentiates it from other specialties within nursing and from other discipline-

1

specific specialties within health informatics. The nursing phenomena of interest are the patient, health, environment, and nurse. Nursing informatics shares interest in these four phenomena, but focuses on the structure and algorithms of data, information, and knowledge used by nurses in their practice (Lange, 1997), whether that practice is clinical, administrative, educational, and/or research centered. Other specialties within nursing are concerned about the content of data and information, and less concerned about the structure of that data and information. Nursing informatics is also charged with ensuring that nursing's data are represented and included in the computerized/electronic processing of health information.

For three decades or more, nurses have held informatics roles and been key stakeholders in developing, implementing, and evaluating informatics solutions. Although implementing informatics solutions continues to be very important, more recently informatics nurse specialists have worked to develop and refine nursing's language, implement telehealth systems, establish NI educational programs, and expand the focus of NI research, among other activities. These examples reflect the diverse nature of NI practice. Because it is difficult to be an expert in each one of these informatics subspecialties, informatics nurse specialists tend to focus their practice in one or two areas of NI. Subsequent discussions in this document that define NI and its practice will expand this concept of differentiated practice.

Defined Research Program

Research within nursing informatics (NI) is exceptionally varied. However, the National Center for Nursing Research (NCNR), within the National Institute for Nursing Research (NINR), identified these specific research priorities for NI. Published by NINR (then the National Center for Nursing Research), the seven priorities for NI research were identified as follows (NCNR, 1993):

- Using data, information, and knowledge to deliver and manage patient care.

- Defining and describing data and information for patient care.

- Acquiring and delivering knowledge from and for patient care.

2

- Investigating new technologies to create tools for patient care.
- Applying patient care ergonomics to the patient–nurse–machine interaction.
- Integrating systems for better patient care.
- Evaluating the effects of nursing informatics solutions.

Most of the recommendations in the 1993 report are impacted by the development of nursing language. In other words, nursing language development and refinement have been seen as a cornerstone of NI research. Therefore, NI research funding has generally been focused in this area.

In 1998, survey results that describe more recent efforts to identify NI research priorities were presented at the international medical informatics meeting (Brennan et al., 1998). A sample of NI researchers across the country was surveyed in 1997 to identify NI research priorities, and to determine how similar or different these priorities were from those established in 1993 by NINR. Ten priorities were identified:

- Standardized language/vocabularies
- Technology development to support practice and patient care
- Data base issues
- Patient use of information technologies
- Using telecommunications technology for nursing practice
- Putting technology into practice
- Systems evaluation issues
- Information needs of nurses and other clinicians
- Nursing intervention innovations for professional practice
- Professional practice issues

In comparing the 1993 NINR report and 1997 survey responses, researchers found a substantial overlap between the two sets of priorities. The greatest emphasis continues to be on nursing language and the development of databases for clinical information. Both sets of priorities also list the need for developing and evaluating decision support tools and evaluating the impact of informatics solutions. Brennan et al. (1998) stated that the newer areas of interest were patients as users of information technology, telecommunications, and issues of privacy and confidentiality.

To date, obtaining funding for NI research in areas other than nursing vocabulary has been difficult. To secure funding, most NI researchers have linked projects to clinical priorities identified by funding agencies. For example, NI researchers could explore funding opportunities at NINR to examine the impact of telehealth systems on patient outcomes. Even though the availability of funding for NI research remains an issue, having a defined research agenda has helped to direct funding agencies and NI researchers. The research agenda has also allowed NI to meet the second required attribute of a specialty.

Organizational Representation

To qualify as a specialty, an area of practice must be represented by at least one organization. Nursing informatics (NI) is well-represented in several organizations at the international, national, regional, and local levels. For example, NI has a work group or special interest group in the American Medical Informatics Association (AMIA); International Medical Informatics Association (IMIA), an international organization; and many regional and local organizations. The NI groups have been essential in (1) establishing the scope of practice and standards of NI, (2) introducing the health informatics community to NI, (3) providing a forum for informatics nurse specialists to network and share issues and solutions, and (4) providing and participating in programs for professional development.

Educational Programs

The first two graduate programs in nursing informatics (NI) were established at the University of Maryland and University of Utah in 1988 and 1990, respectively. Both programs were funded by grants from the Division of Nursing, Health Resources and Services Administration (National Advisory Council on Nurse Education and Practice, 1997). From 1992 to 1998, changes in Title VIII legislation prevented federal funding of NI graduate programs. Because of funding restrictions, development of additional NI educational programs was slowed, but the emergence of NI programs has increased dramatically in the last few years. There is also an increasing interest in developing certificate programs that enable nurses who hold a master's degree to complete special course work in NI.

Some nurses have chosen to enter health informatics, medical informatics, or business programs to acquire needed informatics skills. The widening availability of degree-granting informatics programs has increased educational opportunities for nurses interested in informatics as a career (Gassert, 2000). Thus, the fourth characteristic of a specialty has been fulfilled.

Credentialing

A fifth attribute needed for acknowledging a professional specialty is the development of a certification mechanism. Scope of practice and standards documents for NI were developed under the direction of ANA in 1994 and 1995. These documents were then used by the American Nurses Credentialing Center (ANCC) as a foundation to develop an examination for nurses to become certified as generalists in NI.

Metastructures, Concepts, and Tools of Nursing Informatics

Metastructures are overarching concepts used in theories and sciences. Currently data, information, and knowledge are the metastructures in NI. Sciences underpinning nursing informatics (NI), concepts and tools from information science and computer science, human–computer interaction and ergonomics concepts, and the phenomena of nursing are also of interest in NI.

Metastructures: Data, Information, and Knowledge

In 1989, Graves and Corcoran published a classic work that describes the study of nursing informatics (NI). The article contributes two major thoughts to NI that will be acknowledged here. The first contribution is an information model that identifies data, information, and knowledge as key components of NI practice. Graves and Corcoran (1989) draw from Blum (1986) to define the three concepts as follows:

5

- *Data* are discrete entities that are described objectively without interpretation,

- *Information* is data that are interpreted, organized, or structured, and

- *Knowledge* is information that is synthesized so that relationships are identified and formalized.

As an example, a single instance of vital signs—heart rate, respiration, temperature, and blood pressure—for a single patient can be considered a set of data. A serial set of vital signs taken over time, placed into a context, and compared is considered information. For example, a dropping blood pressure, increasing heart rate, respiratory rate, and fever in an elderly, catheterized patient is recognized as being outside the norm for this type of patient. The recognition that this patient may be septic and needs certain nursing and medical interventions reflects information synthesis (knowledge) based on nursing knowledge and experience.

Figure 1 builds on the work of Graves and Corcoran by providing a depiction of the relationship of data, information, and knowledge. As data are transformed into information and information into knowledge, each level increases in complexity and requires greater application of human intellect. There are multiple feedback loops among the three concepts of data, information, and knowledge. The circles overlap purposefully because the precise distinction among these three concepts becomes blurred at their borders.

Data, which are processed to information and then knowledge, may be obtained from individuals, families, communities, and populations. Data, information, and knowledge are of concern to nurses in all areas of practice. For example, data derived from direct care of an individual patient are described in the previous scenario. Data may then be compiled across patients and aggregated for decision-making by nurse administrators. Further aggregation may address communities and populations. Nurse-educators may create case studies using these data, and nurse-researchers may access aggregated data for systematic study.

The concepts of nursing data, information, and knowledge resonated with informatics nurse specialists and others in the nursing community. The Graves and Corcoran (1989) work was widely cited by others.

6

Figure 1. Transformation of Data to Knowledge.

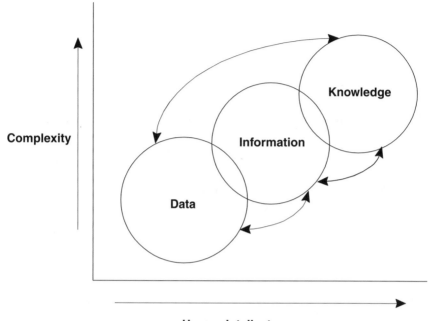

In a later work, the concepts of data, information, and knowledge are more clearly identified as a conceptual framework for the study of NI (Graves et al., 1995). Applying more current terminology, the Graves and Corcoran elements of data, information, and knowledge are part of the metastructure of nursing informatics, meaning that these elements are overarching concepts for the specialty of NI.

Nurses have been recognized as primary processors of information for over 30 years (Jydstrup and Gross, 1966; Zielstroff, 1981). In fact, Jydstrup and Gross estimated that nurses in acute care spent 30% to 40% of their time in information processing activities in the 1960s. Given the significant increases in the rate of data and information generation, it is likely that nurses currently spend even more time managing information.

In more recent years, the concept of nurses as information managers has been expanded to the idea that nurses are knowledge workers. *Knowledge work* is described by Drucker (1993) as nonrepetitive, nonroutine work consuming considerable levels of cognitive activity.

7

WILLIAM F. MAAG LIBRARY
YOUNGSTOWN STATE UNIVERSITY

Knowledge workers use analytical and theoretical knowledge in sophisticated ways and develop complex manual skills. Thus, knowledge workers are often specialists. Business literature discusses knowledge as the basic means of production in contemporary organizations and that organizations are staffed by teams of knowledge workers (Drucker, 1993). Sorrells-Jones and Weaver (1999) state that these concepts are not yet widespread within health care, but clearly nurses and other providers fit the definition of a knowledge worker.

Nurse knowledge workers require support from informatics solutions for at least these processes: (a) storing clinical data, (b) translating clinical data to information, (c) linking clinical data and domain knowledge, and (d) aggregating clinical data (Snyder-Halpern, Corcoran-Perry, and Narayan, 2001). Currently, informatics solutions better support the first two processes. Therefore, it is critical that NI attends to the needs of nurses as knowledge workers by optimizing information technology support for all four processes.

Sciences Underpinning Nursing Informatics

The second contribution of Graves and Corcoran (1989) is a definition of nursing informatics (NI) that has been widely accepted in the field. It states that NI is a combination of nursing science, information science, and computer science to manage and process nursing data, information, and knowledge to facilitate the delivery of health care. Their central notion is that the application of these three core sciences—information science, computer science, and nursing science—is what makes NI unique and differentiates it from other informatics specialties.

In addition to these three core sciences, other sciences may be required to solve informatics issues. For instance, if an informatics nurse specialist is interested in the support of clinical decision-making, then cognitive science may be crucial to weave in with the core sciences. On the other hand, if the informatics nurse specialist is dealing with a system's implementation in an institution, an understanding of organizational theory may be much more pertinent to include in the informaticist's repertoire. Likewise, those studying nursing vocabularies would be wise to have a full understanding of linguistics. Because each informatics nurse specialist must tailor the theoretical support to their area of interest or subspecialty, many sci-

8

ences may be appropriate to add to the core of information, computer, and nursing sciences.

Although the core sciences underpin the work in NI, the practice of the specialty is considered an applied rather than a basic science. The combination of sciences creates a unique blend that is greater than just the sum of its parts, a unique combination that creates the definitive specialty of NI. Further, informatics realizes its full potential within health care when it is grounded within a discipline; in this case, nursing. Computer and information science alone do little if they are not applied to a discipline. Through application, informatics can solve critical information management issues of concern to a discipline.

Concepts and Tools from Information Science and Computer Science

Informatics tools and methods from computer and information sciences are considered fundamental elements of nursing informatics (NI), including:

• Information technology

• Information structures

• Information management and communication

Information technology includes computer hardware, software, communication, and network technologies, which are derived primarily from computer science. The other two concepts are derived primarily from information science. First, *information structures* organize data, information, and knowledge for processing by computers. Second, *information management and communication* is an elemental process within informatics. This basic process is facilitated by information technology that distinguishes informatics from more traditional methods of information management. Thus, NI incorporates three more concepts: information technology, information structures, and the management and communication of information. Underpinning all of these are human–computer interaction concepts.

Human–Computer Interaction and Ergonomics Concepts

Human–computer interaction (HCI) and ergonomics concepts are fundamental concerns for the informatics nurse specialist. Essen-

9

tially, HCI deals with people and computers and the ways they influence each other (Dix et al., 1998). This area blends psychology and/or cognitive science, applied work in computer science (Patel and Kaufman, 1998), sociology, and information science into the design, development, purchase, implementation, and evaluation of applications. For example, an informatics nurse specialist would assess an application before purchase to see if the application design complements the way nurses cognitively process a medication order. A related concept is usability or specific issues of human performance during computer interactions within a particular context (Rubin, 1994). Usability issues address the efficiency and effectiveness of an application (e.g., the ease of learning an application, the ease of using an application, or the speed and errors committed during application use) (Staggers, In press).

The term *ergonomics* is typically used in the United States to focus on the design and implementation of equipment, tools, and machines related to human safety, comfort, and convenience (Langendoen and Costa, 1994). In computing environments, ergonomics concepts commonly refer to attributes of physical equipment, and might be used to optimally arrange workstations and chairs to promote work in an intensive care unit, for example.

HCI, usability, and ergonomics are related concepts. All have as their goal the design of information, information technology, and equipment to promote optimal task completion. Although health care has been slow to embrace the use of HCI concepts, these concepts are essential for creating, selecting, implementing, and evaluating information structures and information technology of use to nurses and patients. Because of their fundamental nature, HCI concepts are listed as a NI assumption and an overarching standard for NI performance later in this document.

Phenomena of Nursing

The phenomena of nursing are the nurse, patient, health, and environment. Actions within nursing are based on the decisions made about these four phenomena. *Decision-making* is the process of choosing among alternatives. The decisions that nurses make can be characterized by both the quality of decisions that must be made and the impact of the actions resulting from those decisions. As knowledge workers, nurses make numerous decisions that affect

10

the life and well-being of individuals, families, and communities. The process of decision-making in nursing is guided by the concept of critical thinking. *Critical thinking* is the intellectually disciplined process of actively and skillfully using knowledge to conceptualize, apply, analyze, synthesize, and/or evaluate data and information as a guide to belief and action (Scriven and Paul, 1997).

Nurses' decision-making includes behaviors, as well as cognitive processes, in an array of decisions, usually surrounding a cluster of issues rather than single decisions. For example, nurses use data transformed into information to determine interventions for patients, families, communities, and populations. Nurses make decisions about potential patient problems and preventive recommendations. They also make decisions based on inter-relationships with others (such as patients, physicians, or social workers) and decisions within specific environments (such as executive offices, classrooms, and research laboratories). In summary, the elements of interest for NI are:

- Data, information, and knowledge

- Nursing science, information science, and computer science

- Nurse, patient, health, and environment

- Decision-making

- Information structures; managing and communicating information and information technology

Terms and Definitions

Although well-established, nursing informatics (NI) is an evolving field that will continue to change rapidly. Definitions and theoretical structures for the specialty have been proposed, but they can be expected to continue to develop over time before stable concepts and definitions are realized.

Terms Used to Label the Role of the Nurse in Informatics

Various terms are in use describing the role of the registered nurse who practices informatics. They include:

- Nurse informaticist

11

- Informatics nurse

- Informatics nurse specialist

- Clinical informaticist

- Informaticist

In this document, the term informatics nurse specialist (INS) is used to encompass all these terms.

The informatics nurse specialist is a registered nurse who is educationally prepared at least at the master's degree level, preferably within nursing. This nurse's graduate level preparation is distinguished by a depth of knowledge of informatics and nursing theory and practice, validated experience in informatics practice, and competence in advanced informatics skills.

Evolution of the Definition of Nursing Informatics

A myriad of definitions have been proposed for nursing informatics (NI) in the past as discussed in Staggers and Thompson (In review). They may be categorized into three areas:

- Technology-focused definitions

- Conceptually focused definitions, and

- Role-oriented definitions

Technology-focused definitions

A definition for NI appeared as early as 1980. Scholes and Barber (1980, p. 70) stated that NI is, "The application of computer technology to all fields of nursing—nursing service, nurse education, and nursing research." Ball and Hannah (1984) modified an early definition of medical informatics, acknowledging that all health care professionals are part of medical informatics. Therefore, NI was defined as "those collected informational technologies which concern themselves with the patient care decision-making process performed by health care practitioners" (p. 3). A year later, Hannah (1985, p. 181) continued the emphasis on technology and added the concept of role within NI in the following definition:

> The use of information technologies in relation to those functions within the purview of nursing, and that are carried out

by nurses when performing their duties. Therefore, any use of information technologies by nurses in relation to the care of their patients, the administration of health care facilities, or the educational preparation of individuals to practice the discipline is considered nursing informatics.

Saba and McCormick (1986) did not specifically use the term NI in their first book, but organized book chapters around computer applications in the four areas of nursing. They defined nursing information systems as systems that use computers to process nursing data into information to support all types of nursing activities or functions.

The emphasis on technology is not limited to early definitions. Zielstorff et al. (1990) also support technology's significance in NI. More recently, Hannah (Hannah, Ball, and Edwards, 1994) and Saba and McCormick (1996) continue to stress the role of technology in NI as it supports the functions of nursing. Hannah et al. continued with her original definition for NI, and Saba and McCormick (1996, p. 226) provided this newer definition:

The use of technology and/or a computer system to collect, store, process, display, retrieve, and communicate timely data and information in and across health care facilities that administer nursing services and resources, manage the delivery of patient and nursing care, link research resources and findings to nursing practice, and apply educational resources to nursing education.

These authors make a salient point about the principal role technology can play in informatics. In fact, for some practitioners, technology is the dominant issue. For others, NI is defined from a more conceptual view.

Conceptually focused definitions

Conceptual approaches to the emerging NI specialty began in the mid-1980s. These approaches gained acceptance in the 1990s.

Schwirian—Schwirian (1986), in a less frequently cited paper, stressed the need for a "solid foundation of NI knowledge, [that] should have focus, direction, and cumulative properties" (p. 134). She emphasized the need for research to be "proactive and model

13

driven rather than reactive and problem-driven" (p. 134). Schwirian cited Hannah's (1985) more technology-oriented definition of NI, but produced a model that expanded thinking beyond just a focus on technology. Her research model outlined a pyramid of users, nursing-related information, goals, and computers (hardware and software) interconnected with bidirectional arrows. Nursing informatics activity lies within the intersection of the other elements. Meant as a stimulus for research in NI, the model could have been used to guide thinking about NI practice as well. The model depicts the inter-relationships among components and includes new concepts of nursing-related information, goals, and context.

Grobe—In 1988, Grobe described nursing informatics as ". . . the application of the principles of information science and theory to the study, scientific analysis, and management of nursing information for purposes of establishing a body of nursing knowledge" (p. 29). This definition was developed by an international team of nurses in the International Medical Informatics Association (IMIA). The timing of the release of this definition may have hindered its adoption because Graves and Corcoran released a paper about the scope of NI shortly thereafter.

Graves and Corcoran—Graves and Corcoran (1989) provided the first widely cited definition of NI, which downplayed the role of technology and incorporated a more conceptually oriented viewpoint:

> A combination of computer science, information science, and nursing science designed to assist in the management and processing of nursing data, information, and knowledge to support the practice of nursing and the delivery of nursing care (p. 227).

This definition broadened the horizon beyond technology. It also provided the first acknowledgment of an information–knowledge link. Graves and Corcoran's definition allowed a concentration on the purpose of technology rather than technology itself. Their transformation of the definition for NI changed the focus from technology to information concepts by expressly incorporating information science as part of the theoretical basis for NI. The centrality of nursing practice in the Graves and Corcoran definition also helps to support the need for NI as a distinct specialty within health informatics.

The 1989 definition was abstracted from earlier work by Graves and Corcoran (1988). The earlier paper placed the concepts of nursing data, decisions, and processes within a theoretical model showing the flow of data, information, and knowledge and the relationships among these key nursing processes. The model described how both research and clinical decision-making impact patient care and serve to build domain knowledge. After identifying the "flow of symbolic content in the discipline of nursing" (p. 172), Graves and Corcoran identified how information system technology could be used to facilitate each of the identified processes and transformations. Interestingly, in the 1989 work the authors removed the context of nursing and de-emphasized the interrelationships among technology, nurse, and patients from their broader model developed in a previous paper. Fewer nurses recognize the fundamental contribution of the earlier paper, as evidenced by the more frequent citation of the 1989 paper (Staggers and Thompson, In review).

Turley—Turley (1996) presents one of the more recent efforts at describing NI. He identified three themes for NI definitions and then proposed a new NI model. Although he analyzed previous definitions of NI, he did not propose a new definition for the field. By focusing on model development, his paper continued a conceptual approach to informatics. Turley's major contribution was adding cognitive science to a model comprised of the original three sciences proposed by Graves and Corcoran (1989). Turley acknowledged the growing interdisciplinary nature of health care and also focused on nursing's unique contributions to informatics.

Role-oriented definitions

At the time of the Graves and Corcoran paper (1989), informatics nurse specialists were becoming more prevalent. The early technology-related definitions suited these individuals because they emphasized the technological aspect of nurses' roles. As NI gained recognition as a nursing specialty, the ANA's Council on Computer

Applications in Nursing (ANA, 1992) provided a new definition for the field. The ANA expanded on the work of others by incorporating the role of the informatics nurse specialist into Graves and Corcoran's earlier definition:

> A specialty that integrates nursing science, computer science, and information science in identifying, collecting, processing, and managing data and information to support nursing practice, administration, education and research; and to expand nursing knowledge. The purpose of nursing informatics is to analyze information requirements; design, implement and evaluate information systems and data structures that support nursing; and identify and apply computer technologies for nursing (ANA, 1992).

The concepts of the systems life cycle first appeared in this definition. Unfortunately, this definition has not been frequently cited in subsequent work (e.g., Henry, 1995; Saba and McCormick, 1996; Turley, 1996).

In 1994, ANA modified its definition in an effort to legitimize the specialty and to guide efforts to create a certification exam. Although the 1994 (ANA) definition continues to provide information on the role of the informatics nurse specialist, the concepts from the systems life cycle are replaced with a more generic discussion of the NI role.

> Nursing informatics is the specialty that integrates nursing science, computer science, and information science in identifying, collecting, processing, and managing data and information to support nursing practice, administration, education, research, and expansion of nursing knowledge. Nursing informatics supports the practice of all nursing specialties, in all sites and settings whether at the basic or advanced level. The practice includes the development of applications, tools, processes, and structures that assist nurses with the management of data in taking care of patients or in supporting their practice of nursing (p. 3).

Although work on NI definitions within the international arena has occurred, this document concentrates on the NI definitions for North America. Given the relative newness of the NI specialty, hav-

16

ing independent thought about definitions is healthy. Then, in the future, international consensus about definitions could occur.

A New Definition for Nursing Informatics

A new definition is needed to address the core elements identified— nurse, patient, health, environment, decision-making and nursing data, information, knowledge, information structures, and information technology. The construct of health is considered to be ubiquitous within nursing, environment, and patients; therefore, this concept is not reiterated within the new definition. Previous definitions underemphasize the role of the patient in informatics, do not mention information communication, and only imply that data and information are used in nurses' decision-making. In particular, the role of patients has dramatically changed in recent years as patients access and evaluate their own health information and become more participative in their own health care decision-making. Recently, nurses have assumed new roles as information brokers and information interpreters.

New Definition for Nursing Informatics

Nursing informatics is a specialty that integrates nursing science, computer science, and information science to manage and communicate data, information, and knowledge in nursing practice. Nursing informatics facilitates the integration of data, information, and knowledge to support patients, nurses, and other providers in their decision-making in all roles and settings. This support is accomplished through the use of information structures, information processes, and information technology.

The Goal of Nursing Informatics

The goal of nursing informatics (NI) is to improve the health of populations, communities, families, and individuals by optimizing information management and communication. This includes the use of technology in the direct provision of care, establishing effective administrative systems, managing and delivering educational experiences, supporting life-long learning, and supporting nursing research.

The Role of the Informatics Nurse Specialist

There are many activities inherent in the role of informatics nurse specialists (Willson, et al., 2000). These nurses typically concentrate on a subset of possible activities. Role activities include, but are not limited to, the following:

- Employ the information systems life cycle and other tools and processes to analyze data, information and information system requirements.

- Design, develop, select, and evaluate information technology, data structures, and decision-support mechanisms into an integrated information system. These systems support patients, nurses and their information management and human-computer interactions within health care contexts.

- Facilitate the creation of nursing knowledge.

In part because of the strong influence that emerging technology has in supporting the work of the informatics nurse specialist, the role is continually evolving. However, the following general roles are identified: project manager, consultant, educator, researcher, product developer, decision support/outcomes manager, and advocate/policy developer. The concept of the informatics nurse specialist as a change agent practicing in interdisciplinary environments is common to all roles.

Project Manager

In the project management role, informatics nurse specialists perform activities that implement the systems life cycle, including: analyzing, designing, developing, selecting, testing, implementing, and evaluating new or modified informatics solutions and data structures that support nursing and the delivery of patient care. The informatics nurse specialist is a catalyst for developing and revising policies and procedures based on system design, workflow reengineering, and input from system users. The project management role combines the skills of communication, change management, process analysis, risk assessment, scope definition, and team building, in conjunction with business and application knowledge in the management of projects involving informatics solutions. Informatics nurse specialists in this role provide input to the organization's strategic plan, evaluate the effectiveness of their projects, and continually strive to improve the quality and efficiency of their informatics solutions.

Consultant

Informatics nurse specialists in the consultant role apply their informatics knowledge and skills to serve as a resource to clients both formally and informally, in external and internal settings. Flexibility, good communication skills, breadth and depth of clinical and informatics knowledge, and excellent interpersonal skills are needed to respond to what can be rapidly changing projects and demands. This diverse role may involve assisting individuals and groups in defining health care information problems and identifying methodologies for implementing, utilizing, and modifying informatics solutions and data structures that support health care access, delivery, and evaluation. A consultant might serve as the project manager for an informatics-related project or may assist the organization's project manager. Consultants may assist clients in writing requests for proposals (RFPs) to elicit vendor bids for informatics solutions and evaluating responses. Other activities may include, but are not limited to, process redesign, strategic/information technology (IT) planning, system implementation, writing informatics publications, reviewing clinical software products, performing market research, and assisting in the planning of conferences, academic, and professional development programs. Nursing informatics consultants may work for a consulting firm, be employed as staff of the organization where they consult, or have an independent consulting practice.

Educator

Education and training are critical components of many nursing informatics (NI) roles and activities, and may directly impact the success or failure of any new/modified informatics solution. Teaching nurses, nursing students, patients, health care consumers, and others about the effective and ethical uses of information technology, as well as NI concepts and theories, is essential for encouraging the optimal use of informatics solutions in nursing practice. Informatics nurse specialists in the educator role develop, implement, and evaluate NI curriculum and educational technologies that meet the educational needs of learners. In this role, educators assess and evaluate NI skills and competencies while providing feedback to learners regarding the effectiveness of the learning activity and the learner's ability to demonstrate newly acquired skills. Educators manage, evaluate, report, and utilize data and information related to learners and the educational delivery system. These informatics nurse specialists are the innovators in defining and developing educational technologies, integrating the solutions into the educational and practice environments, and challenging the systems and organizations to consider and embrace innovative informatics processes and solutions.

Researcher

Informatics nurse specialists in the researcher role conduct the research that underlies the design, development, implementation, and impact of informatics solutions. This includes, but is not limited to:

- Basic research on symbolic representation of nursing phenomena
- Basic research on clinical decision-making in nursing
- Applied research in development of prototype systems
- Patients' use of information tools and resources for health information
- Effective methods for information systems implementation
- Human factors or ergonomics research about the design and impact of systems on patients, nurses, and their interactions
- Evaluation research on the effects of systems on the processes and outcomes of patient care
- Usability testing of applications

For example, conducting research to develop and refine standardized nursing languages is essential in defining, describing, and evaluating data, information, and knowledge relative to patient care. Other examples of NI research might include determining organizational attributes facilitating implementation success, investigating the impact and efficacy of hardware and software informatics solutions, linking nursing interventions to outcomes in large data sets, or determining effective nurse–patient interactions in telehealth contexts. Informatics nurse specialist researchers conduct research using systematic methods of inquiry, including traditional research techniques and newer techniques such as data mining or searching data in informatics solutions and data repositories.

Product Developer

Informatics nurse specialists are assuming expanded roles in the marketing, development, and support of systems software and hardware. In this role, informatics nurse specialists participate in the process of designing, developing, and marketing quality informatics solutions for nurses. Understanding the information needs of nurses, nursing, and patient care, as well as knowledge of business, client services, projected market directions, product design, product development methods, market research, contemporary programming, and modeling language are essential for practicing in a product development role.

Decision Support/Outcomes Manager

As aggregate data are made available from systems, they are used by informatics nurse specialists in a decision support/outcomes management role. Outcomes may be related to any area of nursing practice—clinical, education, research, or administration. For example, outcomes may be determined for patients, families, populations, and institutions. Nurses in this role use system tools to maintain data integrity and reliability, facilitate data aggregation and analysis, identify outcomes, and develop performance measurements. Performing in this role enables nurses to contribute to the development of a knowledge base consisting of the data, information, theories, and models that are used by nurses in decision-making and managing nursing-related problems.

Advocate/Policy Developer

The role of the informatics nurse specialist in advocacy and health policy development continues to expand. Informatics nurse specialists are key to infrastructure development of health policy; that is, knowing the data and information content, the structure of data, and the informatics solutions with those attributes. Informatics nurse specialists are experts in defining the data needed and the structure, management, and availability of those data for decision-making, and as such they advocate for patients, clients, providers, and the enterprise. Policy development may be at any level—a work center, institution, state, national, or international. Role activities include advocating for the ethical use of data and information, evaluating, developing, writing, and implementing policies. Regardless of the level or activity, informatics nurse specialists are active partners in the development of health policy, particularly related to information management and communication, confidentiality and security, patient safety, infrastructure development, and economics.

Other Roles of the Informatics Nurse Specialist

New roles for the informatics nurse specialist have emerged. For example, informatics nurse specialists may be entrepreneurs developing products, relevant content, or the user interface for consumer informatics (Web sites). Other roles may include executive-level positions such as chief information officer (CIO) in provider and vendor organizations, managing an independent practice, or owning a business as a health database designer. Clearly, in the future new roles will continue to evolve.

Tenets of Nursing Informatics

- Nursing informatics is a distinct area of specialty practice within nursing. It has a unique body of knowledge, formal preparation within the specialty, and identifiable techniques and methods.

- Nursing informatics includes both a clinical practice and non-clinical area of practice.

- Nursing informatics supports the efforts of nurses to improve the quality of care and the welfare of health care consumer. Information or informatics methods alone do not improve patient care; rather, this information is used by clinicians and managers to effect improvements in care, information management and patient outcomes.

- Although concerned with information technology, nursing informatics focuses on delivering the right information to the right person at the right time.

- Human factors (human–computer interaction [HCI], ergonomics, and usability) concepts are interwoven throughout the practice of NI.

- Nursing informatics' key concerns include ensuring the confidentiality and security of health care data and information and advocating privacy.

- Nursing informatics promotes innovative, emerging, and established information technologies.

- Nursing informatics collaborates with and is closely linked to other health-related informatics specialties.

The Boundaries of Nursing Informatics

This section discusses what nursing informatics (NI) is and is not. It also summarizes the differences between NI and other specialties in nursing. To reiterate, nursing informatics is a specialty that integrates nursing science, computer science, and information science to manage and communicate data, information, and knowledge in nursing practice. Nursing informatics facilitates the integration of data, information, and knowledge to support patients, nurses, and other providers in their decision-making in all roles and settings. This support is accomplished through the use of information structures and information technology.

Nursing Informatics Differentiated From Other Nursing Specialties

The difference between NI and other nursing specialties is the melding of informatics concepts, tools, and methods with nursing. It is the integration of informatics tools and methods, such as information structure, information technology, information management and communication that distinguish NI. However, we should not confuse what computers can do with the essence of the work at hand. The work of nursing is at the heart of NI and informatics tools and methods only facilitate this work.

23

Although some outside the specialty might consider NI synonymous with information technology, focusing on technology alone does not define NI. Whereas information technology is used extensively within the specialty, information technology is a tool to support the principal concern of NI: nursing information management and communication. Thus, the data and information are central to NI; information technology assists in the optimal management and communication of nursing information.

Information is central to the practice of nursing and all nurses must be skilled in managing and communicating information. However, nurses outside NI are primarily concerned with the *content* of that information, whereas informatics nurse specialists focus on the design, structure, and presentation of information and how these issues impact nurses' decision-making. Table 1 distinguishes the foci of nursing and NI.

Informatics Competencies

Although this document focuses on the informatics nurse specialist, informatics competencies are needed by all nurses whether or not they specialize in nursing informatics. As nursing settings become ubiquitous computing environments, all nurses must be both information and computer literate. Competencies are described for two levels of nurses not schooled in informatics (beginning and experienced nurse) and a third level for the nurse prepared in informatics (Staggers, Gassert, and Curran, 2001). The scope and depth of knowledge in informatics increases with each level from beginning nurse to informatics nurse specialist. Also, each level of competency builds on the previous one. Therefore, before becoming an informatics nurse specialist, the nurse is expected to have demonstrated proficiency in the competencies outlined in the beginning and experienced nurse competency levels. Informatics competencies for nurses may be organized into computer skills, information literacy skills, and overall informatics competencies.

Beginning Nurse

The beginning nurse is a nurse preparing for initial entry into nursing practice or who has just begun a nursing career. This nurse is

Table 1. Comparison of Metastructures, Concepts, and Tools of Nursing and Nursing Informatics

Nursing Focus	Nursing Informatics Focus
Nurses, patients, health, environment	Nursing data, information, and knowledge
Content of information	Design, structure, and presentation of information as it impacts nurses' decision-making
Using information applications and technology	Optimizing information structures, applications, and technology for use in managing and communicating data, information, and knowledge

expected to have fundamental information management and computer literacy skills. Beginning nurses use existing informatics solutions and available information to manage their practice.

Computer literacy skills

Computer literacy is a set of skills that allow individuals to use computer technology to accomplish tasks. These include, but are not limited to, basic computer technology skills such as using a word processor, database, spreadsheet, or using applications to document patient care or communicate via e-mail. These skills are necessary for all nurses, but not sufficient for informatics nurse specialists. Thus, a nurse who takes classes focused on learning applications such as word processing or presentation graphics may be considered computer literate, but is not an informatics nurse specialist.

Information literacy skills

Information literacy is a set of abilities allowing individuals to recognize when information is needed and to locate, evaluate, and use that information appropriately (Association of Colleges and Research Libraries [ACRL], 2000). The primary focus of information literacy is on information access and evaluation. Examples are performing bibliographic retrieval and retrieving and evaluating information from Internet sources. These relevant skills are primarily derived from library science. According to the ACRL, an information literate individual is able to:

- Determine the extent of information needed.

- Access the needed information effectively and efficiently.

- Evaluate information and its sources critically.

- Incorporate selected information into one's knowledge base.

- Use information effectively to accomplish a specific purpose.

- Understand the economic, legal, and social issues surrounding the use of information, and access and use information ethically and legally (ACRL, 2000, p. 2).

Overall informatics competencies

The following overall informatics competencies are required of beginning nurses, those individuals first learning about or entering into nursing practice. Overall informatics activities may include but are not limited to:

- Identifying, collecting, and recording data relevant to the nursing care of patients.

- Analyzing and interpreting patient and nursing information as part of the planning for the provision of nursing services.

- Using informatics applications designed for the practice of nursing.

- Implementing public and institutional policies related to privacy, confidentiality, and security of information. These include patient care information, confidential employer information, and other information gained in the nurse's professional capacity.

Experienced Nurse

Experienced nurses have proficiency in one or more domains of interest. This nurse is highly skilled in information management and communication. Experienced nurses have information and computer literacy skills to support their major area of practice. These nurses see relationships among data elements, and make judgments based on trends and patterns within these data. Experienced nurses use current informatics solutions, but also collaborate with the informatics nurse specialist to suggest improvements to these informatics solutions (Staggers, Gassert, and Curran, 2001). In addition to competencies for beginning nurses, experienced nurse activities include at least the following:

- Use system applications to manage data, information, and knowledge within their specialty area.

- Participate as a content expert to evaluate information and assist others in developing information structures and systems to support their area of nursing practice.

- Promote the integrity of and access to information to include, but not limited to, confidentiality, legal, ethical, and security issues.

- Being actively involved in efforts to improve information management and communication (e.g., supports the development and use of standardized nursing languages).

- Act as an advocate or leader for incorporating innovations and informatics concepts into their area of specialty.

Informatics Nurse Specialist

The informatics nurse specialist is expected to have the competencies outlined in the beginning and experienced nurse competency levels. Moving beyond computer skills, information literacy skills, and overall informatics competencies, the informatics nurse specialist demonstrates the competencies reflected in the standards of practice and professional performance (see pages 32 and 40).

The Interdisciplinary Nature of Nursing Informatics

Nursing informatics is a practice specialty and an applied science. Informatics nurse specialists frequently collaborate with other informaticists to optimize nursing information management and communication. To effect information management and communication, NI may use concepts from many sources besides the three core sciences, which may include, but are not limited to, linguistics, cognitive science, engineering, managerial science, and educational theories.

The practice of NI can be, and often is, within interdisciplinary environments. In fact, most informatics nurse specialists function in interdisciplinary environments, working collaboratively with others in team-oriented or patient-centered work processes. However, the central issues of concern to the specialty of NI are embedded within the discipline itself—data, information, and knowledge used for nurses' decision-making in any environment, in any nursing specialty. Although the work of informatics nurse specialists is typically within interdisciplinary teams, informatics nurse specialists add a nursing voice to these interdisciplinary environments and often ensure that nurses' requirements are adequately addressed within these contexts.

The difference between NI and other informatics specialties rests with NI's focus on the information management and communication of nursing data, information, and knowledge. NI has many elements in common with other informatics specialties; for example, informatics tools methods and concepts from information and computer science. Therefore, the boundaries between nursing informatics and other informatics specialties are not rigid, but dynamic and fluid, allowing for information processing to occur beyond just this one informatics specialty.

Ethics in Nursing Informatics

Nursing's long history includes primary concern for the patient or client and commitment to the professional code of ethics for nurses. Therefore, the *Code of Ethics for Nurses* (ANA, 2001) serves as a framework for the informatics nurse specialist who faces ethical issues and ethical dilemmas. This concern for both the patient and commitment to the Code form the foundation for the informatics nurse specialist's unique expertise and insight in this area.

Although the informatics nurse specialist may not be functioning as a clinician, the issues of confidentiality, security, and privacy surrounding the patient, clinician, and enterprise and the associated data, information, and knowledge are of paramount concern. These issues provide significant opportunities to the information nurse specialist for ethical analysis, decision-making, and subsequent action. For example, the explosion of the human genetic mapping and testing technologies is creating valuable new insights into disease identification and treatment opportunities. However, this also produces potentially damaging outcomes if that same information is incorrectly reported or inadequately safeguarded and becomes available to the wrong person or agency. The informatics nurse specialist in this environment has a responsibility to advocate for confidentiality, data integrity and security, quality management of information, and appropriate decision-making.

More powerful information technologies permit new computing approaches and greater data aggregation and linkage capabilities. But as these opportunities expand, the correct application of the methodologies needs continuing evaluation and monitoring. To ensure that appropriate informatics solutions are implemented, the informatics nurse specialist is instrumental in posing questions, such as:

- Has informed consent of the health care consumer been adequately secured?

- Are the databases protected from external and internal compromise?

- Have the appropriate retention and disposition policies been established?

- Are data information management policies enforced?

- Can client anonymity be maintained?

- Are technical, consultant, and vendor personnel accountable for adherence to security and confidentiality mandates?

- Is the researcher accountable for adherence to security and confidentiality mandates?

- Does the Institutional Review Board (IRB) include examination of the information and database management strategies during the review process to ensure adequate protection of the individual subject, the researcher, and the organization?

Health care professionals are accustomed to adhering to a professional code of ethics. Others in the information management and information systems environments may not embrace such a tradition. Ethical questions or issues arise when common corporate business practices run counter to the ethical mandates of health care professionals. The informatics nurse specialist brings an integrated, systems perspective to discussions of the ethical issues posed by such questions as:

- Is a code of ethics integrated into the expanding distributed environment of Internet health information and health care service delivery?

- What standards are in place to address concerns about conflict of interest when health information resources are posted as part of an organization's or company's marketing strategy?

- Is the individual responding to the e-mail or Internet site query truly a qualified clinician appropriately licensed to practice?

- Are appropriate safeguards in place to protect the sender's identity and privacy, the content and integrity of messages, and the respondent's identity?

The Future of Nursing Informatics

After the Graves and Corcoran (1989) article, others proposed adding the concept of wisdom to the triad of data, information, and knowledge (Nelson and Joos, 1989). *Wisdom* may be defined as the appropriate use of data, information, and knowledge in making decisions and implementing nursing actions. It includes the ability to integrate data, information, and knowledge with professional values when managing specific human problems.

Some nursing informatics (NI) experts believe strongly that wisdom is the purview of humans and cannot or should not be considered as a function within technology. Others believe that informatics solutions consistent with professional values and useful to expert nurses will require the incorporation of wisdom. This controversy makes the inclusion of wisdom into the triad of data, information, and knowledge currently an unresolved issue within NI.

This document represents the state of nursing informatics. However, a number of trends in the field of informatics are currently evident and are mentioned here:

- Ubiquitous computing is becoming a reality and the continued innovation and miniaturization of technology is evident. Consequently, partnering between nurses in all specialties and new technologies is becoming imperative.

- Technological innovations are challenging many traditional processes within health care.

- Telecommunications technologies are one set of tools used in nursing practice.

- Core competencies across informatics specialties should be identified in the near future. Therefore, the distinctions among informatics specialties will continue to blur.

- The speed of information transfer and the increasing availability of communications technologies will impact nurses and informatics nurse specialists in the future, making nursing practice and NI, in particular, more international in practice with worldwide standards, competencies, and curricula.

This section outlined the scope of practice for informatics nurse specialists. In the next section, the standards of practice and professional performance for informatics nurse specialists are addressed.

INFORMATICS NURSE SPECIALIST
STANDARDS OF PRACTICE

Nursing informatics is the specialty that integrates nursing science, computer science, and information science to manage and communicate data, information, and knowledge in nursing practice. Nursing informatics facilitates the integration of data, information, and knowledge to support patients, nurses, and other providers in their decision-making in all roles and settings. This support is accomplished through the use of information structures, information processes, and information technology.

The goal of NI is to improve the health of populations, communities, families, and individuals by optimizing information management and communication. This includes the use of technology in the direct provision of care, in establishing effective administrative systems, in managing and delivering educational experiences, in supporting life-long learning, and in supporting nursing research.

The standards of practice for the informatics nurse specialist are organized around a general problem-solving framework that closely resembles the familiar nursing process of assessment, diagnosis, identification of outcomes, planning, implementation, and evaluation. The problem-solving framework supports all facets of informatics practice, including those without technology, and all areas of nursing practice. Informatics nurse specialists and other informaticians use a structured problem-solving method to identify and clarify issues and select, develop, implement, and evaluate informatics solutions. These steps are not mutually exclusive and topics may overlap multiple identified steps.

Informatics solution is a generic term used in this document to describe the product an informatics nurse specialist recommends after identifying and analyzing an issue. An informatics solution may encompass technology and nontechnology products such as developing a database, purchasing a new computer application, creating nursing vocabulary, designing informatics curricula, creating a spreadsheet, tailoring an application to a particular environment, designing a research study to describe required informatics competencies, describing information flow in a process redesign, or creating a structure for information presentation.

Several overarching standards inherent in every aspect of practice begin the discussion of the informatics nurse specialist standards of practice.

Overarching Standards of Practice for the Informatics Nurse Specialist

The informatics nurse specialist:

1. Incorporates theories, principles, and concepts from appropriate sciences into informatics practice. Examples of theories could include information, systems, and change theories. Principles and concepts could include project management, implementation methods, organizational culture, and database structures.

2. Integrates ergonomics and human–computer interaction (HCI) principles into informatics solution design, development, selection, implementation, and evaluation.

3. Systematically determines the social, legal, and ethical impact of an informatics solution within nursing and health care.

Standard I. Identify the Issue or Problem

The informatics nurse specialist synthesizes data, information, and knowledge to clarify informatics issues or problems.

Measurement Criteria

The informatics nurse specialist:

1. Conducts a needs assessment to refine the issue or problem.

    a. Analyzes current practice, workflow, and the potential impact of an informatics solution on that workflow.

    b. Involves crucial stakeholders in an issue or problem and its informatics solution.

c. Evaluates obtained information and findings for their pertinence to the informatics issue or problem.

d. Integrates current and future requirements into a vision for an informatics solution.

2. Incorporates principles and methods of recognized methodologies, such as structured systems analysis, into problem or issue identification.

3. Uses systematic methods to determine user and technical requirements for informatics issues.

4. Interprets the capabilities and limitations of legacy systems in integration planning and requirements determination.

5. Interprets current legislation, trends, and research affecting health information management.

6. Actively participates in strategic planning.

7. Conducts a market analysis for an informatics solution.

Standard II. Identify Alternatives

The informatics nurse specialist analyzes multiple approaches/ solutions to the informatics issue or problem.

Measurement Criteria

The informatics nurse specialist:

1. Uses problem-solving tools and processes to identify and evaluate approaches and solutions to informatics issues and/or problems. These activities may include:

   a. Conducting a systems analysis to determine information needs.

   b. Developing functional and technical specifications based upon identified needs.

   c. Developing business process redesign recommendations.

   d. Analyzing costs and potential return on investment (ROI) as a basis for selecting and implementing informatics solutions.

e. Judging the fit of the proposed informatics solution with the strategic plan.

2. Uses analytical models to identify and evaluate approaches and solutions to informatics issues and/or problems. These activities may include:

a. Developing conceptual, external, and internal models for representing information needs.

b. Designing models of informatics solutions.

3. Prepares documents to describe information needs for the proposed informatics solution. These activities may include:

a. Developing informal and formal requests for an informatics solution such as a request for information or an RFP.

b. Preparing a response to a request for a proposed informatics solution.

c. Using models to communicate to key stakeholders.

Standard III. Choose and Develop a Solution

The informatics nurse specialist develops an informatics solution for a specific issue or problem.

Measurement Criteria

The informatics nurse specialist:

1. Interprets capabilities and limitations of hardware and software and their relationship to the outcomes of proposed informatics solutions in health care.

2. Incorporates usability testing methods in choosing, developing and evaluating an informatics solution.

3. Analyzes economic, technical, and human resources available to support the informatics solution.

4. Incorporates established informatics standards into the informatics solution.

5. Selects an informatics solution by applying selection criteria appropriate for the targeted users and expected outcomes.

6. Develops an evaluation plan for the informatics solution including measurable outcomes and/or terminal objectives.

7. Develops an informatics solution such as designing a documentation tool, determining clinical vocabulary, tailoring an application to a specific environment, or writing a manuscript about an informatics topic.

8. Actively participates in contract development and negotiations, as appropriate.

Standard IV. Implement the Solution

The informatics nurse specialist manages the process for implementing the solution to the informatics issue or problem.

Measurement Criteria

The informatics nurse specialist:

1. Applies principles and concepts of project management to the implementation of the solution.

2. Demonstrates methods of effective project management when implementing the solution.

3. Demonstrates expertise as a project manager.

4. Designs strategies for effective funding of informatics solutions, which may include:

   a. Developing a budget plan for the procurement of resources and maintenance of an informatics solution.

   b. Determining priorities for requirements within budget constraints.

   c. Employing persuasive communication and political astuteness in funding strategies.

5. Develops policies, procedures, and guidelines based on research and analytical findings, which may include:

a. Supporting the implementation, use, and on-going maintenance of an informatics solution.

b. Ensuring the validity and integrity of data.

c. Promoting health and safety within the particular environment.

d. Ensuring the use of an effective informatics solution.

e. Ensuring the ethical use of informatics solution.

f. Ensuring the confidentiality and security of data and privacy for individuals.

6. Ensures that the informatics solution is in compliance with recognized standards from accrediting and regulatory agencies.

7. Manages strategies for implementing the informatics solution.

8. Applies performance or systems testing methodologies to all phases of implementation of the solution, which may include:

a. Developing procedures, policies, protocols, and scenarios for acceptance testing, conversions, and interface testing.

b. Developing a plan for testing implementation conversion and backup procedures.

c. Developing baseline criteria for system acceptance.

d. Recommending solutions for problems and impediments identified during performance/system testing.

9. Manages education activities for the informatics solution, which may include:

a. Developing an education plan based on measurable, learner-oriented outcomes.

b. Producing education materials based on educational principles.

c. Implementing educational activities for learners.

d. Using innovative educational techniques such as computer-based training or virtual reality as appropriate to learner populations and the specific informatics solution.

e. Evaluating all aspects of educational activities.

10. Applies knowledge of product design, information technologies, and client services to internal and external marketing activities to facilitate the adoption of the solution.

Standard V. Evaluate and Adjust Solutions

The informatics nurse specialist evaluates all processes and solutions used to address the informatics problem.

Measurement Criteria

The informatics nurse specialist:

1. Uses a variety of methods to evaluate the structure, process, and outcome of the informatics solution, which may include:

   a. Assessing the ROI.

   b. Conducting a benefits realization analysis at appropriate intervals during and after solution implementation.

   c. Using summative and formative techniques for a comprehensive evaluation approach.

   d. Using reliable and valid instruments to measure user satisfaction with the implemented informatics solution.

   e. Identifying the extent to which the project budget and schedule are met.

2. Analyzes the impact of the informatics solution on individuals, families, communities, and institutions affected by the solution, which may include:

   a. Adapting market analysis tools and techniques to identify recommended changes to the informatics solution.

   b. Using reliable and valid measures to analyze perceived and actual responses to the informatics solution.

   c. Creating written plans for ongoing analysis of the informatics solution's impact.

3. Disseminates results of evaluation to colleagues, stakeholders and others.

4. Reviews all prior steps in the problem-solving process and makes recommendations, which may include:

    a. Systematically assessing the quality and effectiveness of the problem-solving process and informatics solution.

    b. Using the results of the quality and effectiveness analysis to make or recommend process or structural changes.

    c. Incorporating the results of evaluations into policy, procedure, or protocol documentation.

    d. Changing educational programs based on findings.

5. Uses multiple methods, disseminates information and knowledge synthesized from evaluation activities.

INFORMATICS NURSE SPECIALIST STANDARDS OF PROFESSIONAL PERFORMANCE

Standard I. Quality of Nursing Informatics Practice

The informatics nurse specialist evaluates the quality and effectiveness of nursing informatics practice.

Measurement Criteria

The informatics nurse specialist:

1. Integrates knowledge of current professional practice standards, laws, and regulations into informatics practice.

2. Performs quality improvement activities, which may include:

    a. Identifying aspects of nursing informatics practice important for quality monitoring.

    b. Evaluating indicators used to monitor quality and effectiveness of nursing informatics practice.

    c. Collecting data to monitor quality and effectiveness of nursing informatics practice using structures developed for that purpose.

    d. Analyzing quality data to identify opportunities for improving nursing informatics practice.

    e. Formulating recommendations to improve nursing informatics practice or outcomes.

    f. Implementing activities to enhance the quality of nursing informatics practice.

    g. Developing, implementing, and evaluating policies and procedures to improve the quality of nursing informatics practice.

    h. Synthesizing information about the existing and emerging standards to apply to the nursing informatics practice.

3. Implements the results of quality activities to initiate changes in nursing informatics practice.

Standard II. Performance Appraisal

The informatics nurse specialist evaluates one's own nursing informatics practice in relation to professional practice standards and relevant statutes and regulations.

Measurement Criteria

The informatics nurse specialist:

1. Engages in and conducts performance appraisal on a regular basis, identifying areas of strengths as well as areas where professional development is needed.

2. Seeks constructive feedback regarding one's own practice.

3. Takes action to achieve goals identified during performance appraisal.

4. Seeks peer review as appropriate.

Standard III. Education

The informatics nurse specialist maintains knowledge and competency that reflects current nursing informatics (NI) practice.

Measurement Criteria

The informatics nurse specialist:

1. Maintains current skills and competencies.

2. Seeks new knowledge and skills appropriate to NI practice through professional development activities.

3. Seeks certification, if applicable.

Standard IV. Collegiality

The informatics nurse specialist contributes to the professional development of peers, informatics colleagues, and others.

Measurement Criteria

The informatics nurse specialist:

1. Shares knowledge and skills with peers and colleagues.

2. Contributes to informatics education of students, peers, and colleagues.

3. Provides constructive feedback regarding others' practice.

4. Promotes understanding and effective use of information management and information technology.

5. Promotes understanding of NI by translating NI concepts and practice to others.

6. Participates on multi-professional teams that evaluate health informatics practice.

7. Recommends changes in health care informatics using results from the evaluation of the quality and effectiveness of NI practice.

Standard V. Ethics

The informatics nurse specialist bases decisions and actions on ethical principles.

Measurement Criteria

The informatics nurse specialist:

1. Practices according to the current *Code of Ethics for Nurses* (ANA, 2001).

2. Develops methods to maintain confidentiality, and security of information, data, and knowledge.

3. Advocates for appropriate use of data, information, and knowledge.

4. Practices in a nonjudgmental and nondiscriminatory manner that is sensitive to human diversity.

5. Practices in a manner that preserves and protects human autonomy, dignity, and rights.

6. Seeks available resources as needed when formulating ethical decisions.

Standard VI. Collaboration

The informatics nurse specialist collaborates with others in the conduct of nursing informatics (NI) practice.

Measurement Criteria

The informatics nurse specialist:

1. Collaborates with patients and clients, families, informatics professionals, and others in informatics activities.

2. Collaborates with faculty in developing, maintaining, and evaluating educational and professional development informatics programs.

3. Collaborates with others in building the NI knowledge base. This may include activities such as publishing, policy development, and/or conducting research.

Standard VII. Research

The informatics nurse specialist contributes to the body of informatics knowledge.

Measurement Criteria

The informatics nurse specialist:

1. Integrates best available evidence into nursing informatics practice.

2. Conducts systematic inquiry of informatics problems and issues.

3. Disseminates information and knowledge related to systematic inquiry.

4. Develops informatics policies, procedures, and guidelines based on systematic inquiry.

5. Formulates an informatics research program.

Standards VIII. Resource Utilization

The informatics nurse specialist considers factors related to safety, effectiveness, cost, and impact in conducting informatics practice.

Measurement Criteria

The informatics nurse specialist:

1. Evaluates factors related to safety, effectiveness, costs, and impact when developing and implementing information management solutions.

2. Applies strategies to obtain appropriate resources for informatics initiatives.

3. Assigns tasks or delegates responsibilities appropriately based on the nursing informatics activity being conducted.

4. Promotes adoption of activities that assist others in becoming informed about costs, risks, and benefits of information management and information technology solutions.

Standard IX. Communication

The informatics nurse specialist employs effective communications.

Measurement Criteria

The informatics nurse specialist:

1. Is fluent in informatics terminology and standardized languages.

2. Articulates informatics requirements to other disciplines.

3. Interprets communication to and from others, such as informatics professionals, clinicians, patients, executives, and vendors.

4. Communicates complex concepts concisely.

5. Demonstrates persuasive abilities in communication.

6. Applies established guidelines to written communication.

GLOSSARY

Beginning nurse—A nurse preparing for initial entry into nursing practice or who has just begun a nursing career.

Data—Discrete entities that are described objectively without interpretation.

Experienced nurse—A nurse with proficiency in one or more domains of interest.

Informatics solution—A generic term used to describe the product an informatics nurse specialist recommends after identifying and analyzing an issue. Informatics solutions may encompass technology and nontechnology products such as information systems, new applications, nursing vocabulary, or informatics curricula.

Information—Data that are interpreted, organized, or structured.

Knowledge—Information that is synthesized so that relationships are identified and formalized.

Nursing informatics (NI)—A specialty that integrates nursing science, computer science, and information science to manage and communicate data, information, and knowledge in nursing practice. Nursing informatics facilitates the integration of data, information, and knowledge to support patients, nurses, and other providers in their decision-making in all roles and settings. This support is accomplished through the use of information structures, information processes, and information technology.

REFERENCES

American Nurses Association (ANA). (2001). *Code of Ethics for Nurses with Interpretive Statements*. Washington, DC: American Nurses Publishing.

————. (1995). *Standards of Practice for Nursing Informatics*. Washington, DC: American Nurses Publishing.

————. (1994). *Scope of Practice for Nursing Informatics*. Washington, DC: American Nurses Publishing.

————. Council on Computer Applications in Nursing. (1992). *Report on the Designation of Nursing Informatics as a Nursing Specialty*. Congress of Nursing Practice unpublished report. Washington, DC: American Nurses Association.

The Association of Colleges and Research Libraries (ACRL). (2000). *Information Literacy Competency Standards for Higher Education*. San Antonio, TX: American Library Association.

Ball, M. J., and K. J. Hannah. (1984). *Using Computers in Nursing*. Reston, VA: Reston Publishing Co.

Blum, B. L. (1986) *Clinical Information Systems*, p. 35. New York: Springer-Verlag.

Brennan, P. F. (1994). The relevance of discipline. *Journal of the American Medical Informatics Association*, 1(2): 200–201.

Brennan, P. F., R. D. Zielstorff, J. G. Ozbolt, and I. Strombom. (1998). Setting a national research agenda in nursing informatics. In B. Cesnik, A. T. McCray, and J. R. Scherrer (eds). *Medinfo '98: Proceedings of the Ninth World Congress on Medical Informatics*, pp. 1188–1191. Amsterdam: IOS Press.

Dix, A., J. Finlay, G. Abowd, and R. Beale. (1998). *Human–Computer Interaction*. London: Prentice Hall Europe.

Drucker, P. F. (1993). *Post Capitalist Society.* New York: Harper Business Publishers.

Gassert, C. A. (2000). Academic preparation for nursing informatics. In Ball, M. J., K. J. Hannah, S. K. Newbold, and J. V. Douglas (eds). (2001). *Nursing Informatics: Where Caring and Technology Meet, 3rd ed.,* pp. 15–32. New York: Springer-Verlag.

Graves, J. R., L. K. Amos, S. Huether, L. Lange, and C. B. Thompson. (1995). Description of a graduate program in clinical nursing informatics. *Computers in Nursing* 13: 60–70.

Graves, J. R., and S. Corcoran. (1989). The study of nursing informatics. *Image* 21(4): 227–231.

———. (1988). Design of nursing information systems. *Journal of Professional Nursing* 4: 168–177.

Grobe, S. J. (1988). Nursing informatics competencies for nurse educators and researchers. In Peterson, H. E., and U. Gerdin-Jelger (eds). *Preparing Nurses for Using Information Systems: Recommended Informatics Competencies,* pp. 25–33. New York: National League for Nursing.

Hannah, K. J. (1985). Current trends in nursing in informatics: Implications for curriculum planning. In Hannah, K. J., E. J. Guillemin, and D. N. Conklin (eds). *Nursing Uses of Computers and Information Science,* pp. 181–187. Amsterdam: North-Holland.

Hannah, K. J., M. J. Ball, and M. J. A. Edwards. (1994). *Introduction to Nursing Informatics.* New York: Springer-Verlag.

Henry, S. (1995). Nursing informatics: State of the science. *Journal of Advanced Nursing* 22: 1182–1192.

Jydstrup, R. A., and J. J. Gross. (1966). Cost of information handling in hospitals. *Health Services Research* 1(3): 235–271.

Lange, L. L. (1997). Informatics nurse specialist: Roles in health care organizations. *Nursing Administration Quarterly* 21(3): 1–10.

Langendoen, D., and D. Costa. (1994). *The Home Office Computer Handbook*. New York: Windcrest/McGraw-Hill.

National Advisory Council on Nurse Education and Practice (NACNEP). (1997). *A National Agenda for Nursing Education and Practice*. Rockville, MD: U.S. Department of Health and Human Services, Health Resources and Services Administration.

National Center for Nursing Research (NCNR). (1993). *Nursing Informatics: Enhancing Patient Care: A Report of the NCNR Priority Expert Panel on Nursing Informatics/National Center for Nursing Research*, pp. 3–9. NIH Publication No. 93-2419. Bethesda, MD: U.S. Department of Health and Human Services.

Nelson, R., and I. Joos. (1989). On language in nursing: From data to wisdom. *PLN Vision* Fall: 6.

Panniers, T. L., and C. A. Gassert. (1996). Standards of practice and preparation for certification. In Mills, M. E., C. A. Romano, and B. R. Heller (eds). *Information Management in Nursing and Health Care*, pp. 280–287. Springhouse, PA: Springhouse Corporation.

Patel, V., and D. Kaufman. (1998). Medical informatics and the science of cognition. *Journal of the American Medical Informatics Association* 5(6): 493–502.

Rubin, J. (1994). *Handbook of Usability Testing: How to Plan, Design, and Conduct Effective Tests*. New York: John Wiley and Sons.

Saba, V. K., and K. A. McCormick. (1996). Nursing informatics. In *Essentials of Computers for Nurses, 2nd ed.* pp. 221–263. New York: McGraw-Hill.

———. (1986). *Essentials of Computers for Nurses*. Philadelphia: J. B. Lippincott.

Scholes, M., and B. Barber. (1980). Towards nursing informatics. In Linberg, D. A. D., and S. Kaihara (eds). *MEDINFO: 1980*, pp. 70–73. Amsterdam Netherlands: North-Holland.

Schwirian, P. (1986). The NI pyramid-A model for research in nursing informatics. *Computers in Nursing* 4(3): 134–136.

Scriven, M., and R. Paul. (1997). A working definition of critical thinking by Michael Scriven and Richard Paul. Available from http://lonestar.texas.net/~mseifert/crit2.html (from the Palo Alto College Critical Thinking Resource Home Page). Accessed September 18, 2001.

Snyder-Halpern, R., S. Corcoran-Perry, and S. Narayan. (2001). Developing clinical practice environments supportive of the knowledge work of nurses. *Computers in Nursing* 19(1): 17–23.

Sorrells-Jones, Jean, and Diana Weaver. (1999.) Knowledge workers and knowledge-intense organizations. Part 1: A. Promising framework for nursing and healthcare. *Journal of Nursing Administration* Jul/Aug; 29(7/8): 12–18.

Staggers, N. (In press). Human-computer interaction in health care organizations. In Englebardt, S., and R. Nelson. *Health Care Informatics: An Interdisciplinary Approach.* St. Louis, MO: Harcourt.

Staggers, N., and C. B. Thompson. (In review). The evolution of definitions for nursing informatics. *Journal of the American Medical Informatics Association.*

Staggers, N., C. A. Gassert, and C. Curran. (2001). Informatics competencies for nurses at four levels of practice. *Journal of Nursing Education* 40(7): 303–316.

Styles, M. M. (1989). *On Specialization in Nursing: Toward a New Empowerment.* Kansas City, MO: American Nurses Foundation.

Turley, J. (1996). Toward a model for nursing informatics. *Image* 28: 309–313.

Wilson, D., G. Bjornstad, et al. (2000) Nursing informatics career opportunities. In Carty, B. (ed). *Nursing Informatics: Education for Practice.* New York: Springer.

Zielstorff, R. (1981). How computer systems influence nursing activities in hospitals. In *The Proceedings of the First National Conference: Computer Technology and Nursing*, pp. 1–6. Bethesda, MD: National Institutes of Health.

Zielstorff, R., L. Abraham, H. Werley, V. K. Saba, and P. Schwirian. (1990). Guidelines for adopting innovations in computer-based information systems for nursing. *Computers in Nursing* 7(5): 203–208.

WILLIAM F. MAAG LIBRARY
YOUNGSTOWN STATE UNIVERSITY